Analyzing
Sports Drinks

What's right for you?

Carbohydrate or Electrolyte Replacement?

D1547144

By
Nina Anderson, S.P.N.
in cooperation with Dr. I. Gerald Olarsch, N.D.

Published by
Safe Goods/ New Century Publishing 2000
Markham, Ontario

Analyzing Sports Drinks

Nina Anderson,
Specialist in Performance Nutrition (S.P.N.)

in cooperation with
Dr. I. Gerald Olarsch,
Naturopathic Doctor

ISBN 1-884820-69-7
Printed in the United States of America

Analyzing Sports Drinks is not intended as medical advice. It is written solely for informational and educational purposes. Please consult a health professional should the need for one be indicated.

Published by Safe Goods/New Century Publishing 2000
60 Bullock Dr., Unit 6, Markham, ON L3P 3P2
(905) 471-5711
US Marketing Office: (413) 229-7935

Table of Contents

Chapter 1: Sports drinks are not all the same.

Sports drinks are everywhere today, being consumed in the workplace, at home, and in the car as well as before, during, and after exercise. They are outperforming other beverage segments as more choices are being offered each day.[1] Several types of sports drinks are being marketed: a) electrolyte replacement drinks, b) carbohydrate replacement drinks, c) combination drinks of electrolytes and carbohydrates. While there may be a place for all within the sports arena, on closer examination, the drinks are used for completely different purposes. Electrolyte replacement drinks are designed to replace the fluids (water) and electrolytes (sodium, potassium, chromium, manganese, etc.) lost during exercise. Carbohydrate drinks are the acceptable choice for instant energy during strenuous exercise and muscle recovery afterwards. Many carbohydrate drinks may also include electrolytes. According to the American College of Sports Medicine, consuming adequate food and fluid before, during, and after exercise can help maintain blood glucose levels during exercise, maximize exercise performance, and improve recovery time. Athletes should be well hydrated before beginning exercise and should also drink enough fluid during and after exercise to balance fluid losses.[2]

Not all sports-minded people need carbohydrate drinks, but most of them need electrolyte replacement. According to the International SportsMedicine Institute, many Americans are dehydrated, even before exercise, because they don't drink enough water. In the United States, dehydration in children results in 200,000 hospitalizations and an estimated 400 deaths per year.[3] The average person normally loses between 3-6 liters from normal bowel and urinary elimination. Moisture is also lost just from breathing. Some of the

---

[1] Bachman, Tom, "The spurt in sports drinks." Beverage Industry, June 2000.

[2] Position of Dietitians of Canada, the American Dietetic Assn., and the American College of Sports Medicine: Nutrition and Athletic Performance. Can J Diet Pract Res 2000, winter; 61(4):176-192.

[3] Duggan, C., R. Glass, M. Santosham, "Oral rehydration therapy in children." Patient Care, April 30, 1992.

more obvious signs of low water levels in your body include headaches and fatigue.

Sports endurance will be compromised if dehydration worsens. Heart rate increases and oxygen (and nutrient delivery to the muscles) can drop 10 percent even with mild exercise like hiking.[4] Unreplaced water losses equal 2 percent of body weight and will impact heat regulation. At 3 percent loss there is a decrease in muscle cell contraction times and when fluid losses equal 4 percent of body weight there is a 5-10 percent drop in overall performance which can last up to four hours. Lost with this fluid are electrolytes and essential minerals. Mineral replacement is essential to helping restore proper blood volume and blood sugar levels, and is necessary for enzymatic reactions that promote proper blood volume. Without them the quality of performance during long-term or explosive short-term exercise decreases.

Trying to get people to drink lots of water is not always easy. Most prefer juice or soda pop. Manufacturers have come to the rescue with many flavored and sweetened sports drinks, but are they all the same? These include unsweetened electrolyte replacement drinks, carbohydrate-electrolyte drinks, carbohydrate and protein drinks, and functional fluids (nutrients added such as vitamins or herbs). Many drinks include high-caloric sugars (glucose, fructose, maltodextrin, cereal starches) as carbohydrates. These are not recommended for dieters or diabetics and may not be beneficial in electrolyte drinks because the added sugar needs to be broken down by the digestive system thus delaying electrolyte absorption. Sports drinks that contain not only water, but also sodium and carbohydrates, do not quench thirst as quickly as water does.[5] When your body wants water, it wants it immediately, and carbohydrates may actually interfere with water absorption.

Research shows that even though the process of stomach emptying is slowed by sugar, the absorption rate in the small

---

[4] Tilton, Buck, "Just Add Water; why powdered "sports" drinks belong in your pack." Backpacker, Feb. 1993, Vol. 21, No.1, p. 16.
[5] Fox, Martha Capwell, "Fluid mechanics." Rodale's Fitness Swimmer, July-August, 1999.

intestine increases when slightly sweetened drinks are consumed. Tests indicate that repeated ingestion of a drink containing carbohydrates in concentrations of not more than 4-8 percent during prolonged exercise does not compromise the rate of gastric emptying.[6] Higher levels of carbohydrates could impair gastric emptying and intestinal absorption of fluids needed by the athlete. Beverage osmolality [absorption] is less important than beverage energy content in influencing gastric emptying rate at these concentrations.[7] This information relates best to absorption of a carbohydrate drink rather than a pure electrolyte drink.

To receive benefit from electrolytes, the body must be able to utilize the minerals. Dr. George Earp-Thomas, research scientist, who along with a team of researchers funded by the Rockefeller Foundation, conducted a worldwide study on soil microbes and minerals. He discovered that when combined, different *inorganic* minerals from decaying rock were not always compatible with each other. He finally added the Foulhorn bacteria, that are found on the surface of mineralized rocks beneath the sea. This allowed the mineral mixture to become stable. He discovered this bacteria would make new compounds, thus transforming the elements into an *organic* mineral compound that could be readily absorbed by the body. He claimed that benefits from the intake of these organic minerals include warding off colds, and changing the constitution of blood so it becomes inhospitable to germs. Other supplement manufacturers supply minerals in the form of plant organics. Minerals in an organic form are best utilized by the body. This is an important consideration when purchasing electrolyte products.

For fast electrolyte replacement it is best to take pure water from a good source (filtered tap water, bottled water, spring water) and add a proper ratio of absorbable electrolyte-forming minerals. Some schools of thought advise adding a small bit of carbohydrate

---

[6] American College of Sports Medicine. "Position Stand: Heat and cold illnesses during distance running." Med. Sci. Sports Exerc. 18:I-x, 1996.

[7] Murray, Robert, William Bartoli, John Stofan, Mary Horn, and Dennis Eddy, "A comparison of the gastric emptying characteristics of selected sports drinks." International Journal of Sport Nutrition, Sept. 1999 p. 263(12).

sweetener to hasten absorption, while others think it hampers absorption.

Formulations with too *many* trace-minerals in combination can actually prevent electrolyte formation because they can compete with one another for absorption. Too few trace-minerals in a drink are unable to form the proper electrolyte balance for the minerals to be able to enter the cell and maximize rehydration.[8] Sports drinks that include sodium and potassium as electrolyte-forming minerals, are primarily included to replace the "salts" removed from the body by sweat during heavy exercise. Sodium, in amounts between 500-700 milligrams per liter, is recommended for prolonged exercise because it may enhance palatability and the drive to drink, therefore increasing the amount of fluid consumed.[9] Most drinks do not contain this level of sodium, therefore, replacement may be necessary for those who are vigorously working their muscles. For people who are dehydrated from a dry environment (such as airplanes or indoor winter climates), or who exercise mildly (kayakers, hikers), lower sodium levels and a drink with a more complete electrolyte complement is recommended.

Sodium in bicarbonate form may actually help to counteract the buildup of lactic acid in the blood during *heavy* exercise. Benefits to athletes include improved anaerobic performance, especially during exercise regimens that are longer and more strenuous in duration.[10] Several studies reported runners using 0.3 gm/kg of sodium bicarbonate with water over a two to three hour period when competing in 400-800 meter events, thereby improving their times by several seconds.[11] As in all supplementation, use moderation. Smaller amounts of sodium bicarbonate may be beneficial, but loading up with large quantities requires exploiting a challenging energy need and, when taken in excess, may cause diarrhea. As in

---

[8] Martlew, Gillian, N.D., *Electrolytes The Spark of Life*, 1998 revised & updated, Nature's Publishing, Murdock FL.

[9] American College of Sports Medicine. "Position Stand: Heat and cold illnesses during distance running." Med. Sci. Sports Exerc. 18:I-x, 1996.

[10] Berning, Jacqueline R., Nelson Steen, Suzanne, *Nutrition for sport and exercise,* Aspen Publishers, Inc. Gaithersburg, MD, 1998.

[11] Williams, M.H., "Bicarbonate loading," Sports Sci Exchange, 1992;4(36).

carbo-loading, it must be considered on an individual basis for specific energy needs.

A major part of the sports drink market is geared towards carbohydrate drinks. Carbohydrates are the considered the principal dietary source of energy. Muscle cells store limited amounts of adenosine triphosphate (ATP), a high-energy phosphogen, and depend upon metabolic pathways to provide sufficient ATP for muscle function during activity. Power events of short duration require the rapid hydrolysis of ATP for energy, which is significantly depleted within10-20 seconds of high-intensity activity, thereby limiting its use as a source for energy.[12] In exercise of longer duration, the source of carbohydrate extraction from the energy pool may shift from the ATP muscle glycogen pool to circulating blood glucose. If blood glucose cannot be maintained, performance will decrease.[13] Fat contributes to the energy pool, but the portion of energy from fat decreases as exercise intensifies.[14] Protein also contributes to the energy pool, but probably provides less than 5 percent of the energy expended although it may contribute to the maintenance of blood glucose.[15]

There is no absolute requirement for dietary carbohydrates, although the brain, red blood cells, and some cells in the kidneys use glucose as a preferred source of energy.[16] The need for carbohydrate ingestion before, during, and after exercise has been

---

[12] Conley, K., "Cellular energetics during exercise," Adv Vet Sci Comp Med. 1994; 38A:1-39.

[13] Coyle, E.F., Coggan, A.R., Hemmert, M.K., Ivy, J.L., "Muscle glycogen utilization during prolonged strenuous exercise when fed carbohydrate." J. Appl. Physiol. 61:165-172, 1986.

[14] Bergman, B.D., Butterfield, G.E., Wolfel, E.E., Casazza, G.A., Lopashuk, G.D., Brooks, G.A., "Evaluation of exercise and training on muscle lipid metabolism." Am.J. Physiol. 176:E106-E117, 1999.

[15] Phillips, S.M., Atkinson, S.A., Tarnopolsky, M.A.,MacDougall, J.D., "Gender differences in leucine kinetics and nitrogen balance in endurance athletes." J. Appl. Physiol. 75:2134-2141, 1993.

[16] Anderson, James W., M.D., J.P. Flatt, Ph.D, Peter, J. Reeds, Ph.D., "Carbohydrates," www.nutrition.org.

obtained from athletic performance studies.[17] Almost everyone agrees that carbohydrate feeding will improve performance in endurance events of moderate intensities over two hours.[18] In practice, athletes are instructed to drink 6-12 oz. of a carbohydrate drink immediately prior to beginning strenuous activity, and continue with additional "dosages" during the exercise (to reduce fatigue) and after (as muscle glucose replacement).[19]

Studies from sports teams show that the intake of carbohydrates is derived from both food and from sports drinks. According to the International Sports Science Association, pre-exercise, exercise, and post-exercise carbohydrate ingestion needs to include fluid and electrolyte requirements. The pre-exercise meal is ideally high in carbohydrates, low in protein, fat, and sugar, and eaten about three hours prior to exercise. This is important because it take this long for the stomach to empty and glucose to enter the bloodstream. Consuming sugar immediately before exercise can increase the risk of GI distress in the form of cramps, nausea, diarrhea, and bloating.

During exercise if a sports beverage is taken and is too high in carbohydrate content (normally glucose or sugar), it will increase the time it takes the stomach to empty.[20] This prolongs the time for absorption.

Replacing the glycogen lost from muscles in the first two hours after exercise is the primary usage for carbohydrates during heavy exercise.[21] Glucose and sucrose are the carbohydrates of

---

[17] Coyle, E.F., Hagberg, J.M., Hurley, B.F., Martin, W.H., Ehsani, A.A., Holloszy, J.O., "Carbohydrate feeding during prolonged strenuous exercise can delay fatigue." J.Appl Physiol. 1983;55:230-235.

[18] Andersen, Douglas, DC, DACBSP, CCN, DACBN, "Sports Nutrition Update – Abstracts from the American college of Sports Medicine 43rd Annual Meeting." Dynamic Chiropractic Online, 2001.

[19] Garrett, Dr. William Jr., Lohnes, John, Kirkendall, Dr. Don, Marchak, Patty, "Hydration. Fluids – Drink Types," Duke University Medical Center and Univ. North Carolina Hospital Sports Medicine Section.

[20] Gastelu, Daniel,M.S., M.F.S., Hatfield, Frederick C., Ph.D. *Weight Control, Fitness, and Performance Nutrition: The Complete Guide*, ISSA, 2000.

[21] Applegate, Liz, "Liquid Assets," Runner's World, July 2000.

choice and considered twice as effective as fructose in restoring muscle glycogen. However, the role of adequate glycogen resources in preventing muscle cramps is speculative and still being debated.

• *New information on carbohydrate replacement.* According to Dr. Zakir Ramazanov, Ph.D., who is one of the foremost biochemists and molecular biologists in the world, there is an alternative for long-term stamina. "Sports and fitness enthusiasts consider carbohydrates the best source of energy, when they actually are a relatively poor source. Glucose is considered a fast, easy source of energy. Fatty acids are the richest source of energy. The use of more energy-rich fatty acids for production is far better than relying on carbohydrates alone. Fatty acids are activated by L-carnitine before they enter into the cells, where these rich-in-energy compounds are metabolized. Liberated energy is eventually used in the product of ATP (the universal source of energy generated by the oxidation of carbohydrates, fat and proteins) and Creatine phosphate (a reservoir of high-energy phosphoryl groups that can eventually accumulate as ATP). In fact, fatty acids play a greater role in supporting the energy demands of the body during *long-term* exercise than glucose alone."[22] During times of high physical activity, energy and macronutrient needs must be met, and fat intake should be adequate to provide essential fatty acids and fat-soluble vitamins for energy. When more fat is burned, less muscle glycogen is used. This "glycogen sparing" effect aids endurance because glycogen stores are limited, but fat stores are abundant.[23]

[22] Ramazanov, Dr. Zakir, Suarez, Dr. Maria del Mar Bernal, *Effective Natural Stress and Weight Management Using Rhodiola Rosea and Rhododendron Caucasicum,* Safe Goods, E. Canaan, CT, 1999.
[23] Berning, Jacqueline R., Nelson Steen, S., *Nutrition for sport and exercise,* Aspen Publishers, Gaithersburg, MD, 1998.

Our diets should provide moderate amounts of energy from fat (20-25 percent of energy).[24] Consuming adequate food and fluid before, during, and after exercise can help maintain blood glucose levels, maximize performance, and improve recovery time. Since most people's diets are fatty acid deficient, it would follow that their structure is more prone to muscle breakdown. Carbo-loading (eating lots of carbohydrates) before a sports event has been a common practice to "shore up" the muscles.

Maintaining a higher fatty-acid base will enforce the muscles without excessive carbo-loading. Dr. Ramazanov suggests supplementing your diet with an herb grown in the mountains of Russia, *Rhodiola rosea*. This herb has shown to raise the levels of fatty acids found in the blood, thereby significantly increasing muscle ATP and creatine phosphate levels. The results of tests on athletes shows enhanced physical performance and increased endurance by accelerating recovery from fatigue when using Rhodiola. [25]

Beginning in the early 1930s research has been conducted on a classification of herbs known as adaptogens. These not only include Rhodiola, but Rhaponticum carthamoides, a natural anabolic steroid that has shown in athletic training situations, to burn fat into muscle up to twenty times faster. It is shown to improve nitrogen retention while increasing protein synthesis at the cellular level and is being used by athletes to improve their physical abilities. Because it contains the phyto-nutrient, ecdysterone, Rhaponticum has shown to increase endurance and rebuild damaged muscles in addition to its ability to synthesize muscle tissue. Supplementing an electrolyte-replacement drink with Rhodiola and Rhaponticum may be a healthier alternative to sports drinks that contain dyes, sugar, or additives.

---

[24] "Position of Dietitians of Canada, the American Dietetic Association, the American College of Sports Medicine: Nutrition and Athletic Performance," Can J Diet Pract Res 1000, Winer; 61(4):176-192.

[25] Saratikov, A.S., Salnik,B.U., Revina, T.A., 1968, "Biochemical Characteristics of the Stimulative Action of Rodosine during prescribed Muscular Workloads. Proceedings of the Siberian Department of Academy of Sciences of the USSR," Biological Sciences, 5:108-115.

Another supplement to enhance ATP production is alpha-ketoglutarate, an intermediate of the citric acid cycle responsible for the basic energy component, ATP. Laboratory studies show in cell cultures that depletion of alpha-ketoglutarate results in loss of available cellular energy because of the decreased formation of ATP. Alpha-ketoglutarate is used as a supplement by some athletes to extend the time to energy depletion. Research is also underway on Glycerol, a 3-carbon nonintoxicating alcohol, a product of triacylglycerol (free fatty acids), which is used in the body's citric acid cycle of aerobic energy metabolism. Glycerol enhances hydration in muscles, thereby reducing fatigue and need for continued carbohydrate ingestion. In studies on athletes, it has shown to increase their total body water by nearly 2.5 percent which helped them adapt to heat during extended exercise.[26] It is the choice of the consumer to pick a product that works for them and tastes good. There is a place for carbohydrate sports drinks as a supplement to electrolyte replacement drinks, but they are not interchangeable. You may use carbohydrate drinks in addition to electrolyte replacement drinks, but at different times in relation to the intended sports activity.

---

[26] Robergs, R.A., et al. "Glycerol biochemistry, pharmacokinetics: clinical and practical applications." Sports Med, 1998, Sep; 26(3) 145-67.

Chapter: **What are electrolytes?**

Electrolyte is a "medical/scientific" term for mineral salts, specifically ions. Electrolytes are the spark that keeps our body running. They are necessary for life. They are important because they are what your cells (especially nerve, heart, muscle) use to maintain voltages across their cell membranes and to carry electrical impulses (nerve impulses, muscle contractions) across themselves and to other cells. [27]

These electro-chemicals influence the body's pH — a chemical balance that determines how effectively the biological systems run. When there is a deficiency of body electricity, body functions slow down and eventually stop. Micronutrients play an important role in energy production, hemoglobin synthesis, maintenance of bone health, adequate immune function, and the protection of body tissues from oxidative damage. They are also required to help build and repair muscle tissue following exercise.

Electrolytes are formed when certain minerals come together in solution and create electrical activity providing energy for the body. When the electrolytes are dissolved, they break apart into charged particles called ions. The ions carry either a negative or positive charge. These charged particles create the electricity. If the minerals are missing, your spark will fizzle.

Electrolytes facilitate delivery of oxygen to achieve and maintain peak brain function and proper nervous system response. The constant firing of micro-electric impulses across the synapses of the brain requires a great deal of energy. Only electrolytes can supply this. If, because of electrolyte imbalance, there isn't enough oxygen available for the nerve cells to fire when needed, the brain functions less effectively. The body uses oxygen to turn nutrients into energy through the process of primary oxigenation. This simply means that electrolytes help the oxygen create a chemical reaction that ultimately allows the body to "burn" the nutrients as fuel. In a nutshell, bio-oxidation liberates energy — which facilitates life.

---

[27] University of Waterloo, Canada website:
http://sciborg.uwaterloo.ca/~cchieh/cact/c120/electrolyte.html.

The direction of health care in the future will depend on finding solutions for the ever-growing mineral deficiencies in our food and water. For those of us who take the bull by the horns, we refuse to wait! Products are available now that effectively give back to the body what is missing. Electrolyte supplementation can effectively recharge your battery and may just be an absolute necessity for future generations.

• *Fish use electrolytes as propellants.*
Gillian Martlew, N.D., author of *Electrolytes The Spark of Life*[28] relates a story where a man watches a fish swim in circles in a particular pool at the base of a waterfall. Round and round he swam until he finally bounded *up* the waterfall. What that fish did was create an electric charge in his body taken from the swirling waters at the base of the tumbling waterfall. With this charge he was able to challenge gravity and swim up the tumbling waters. This story lets us know how important the vortex of energy in water can be. Our ancestors used to become invigorated by drinking from rushing mountain brooks. Today most water is filtered or mineral deficient reducing its electrolyte content. In most cases, especially when exercising, we must add an electrolyte drink or supplement to our diet to recharge our *spark*!

---

[28] Martlew, Gillian, N.D., *Electrolytes The Spark of Life*, 1998 revised & updated, Nature's Publishing, Murdock FL.

Chapter 3: **Electrolyte/mineral supplementation.**

When the human body is electrolyte deficient, vital nutrients are not oxidized effectively enough. This compromises the body's ability to get the fuel it needs to run at peak performance and to fight disease. Sports enthusiasts know the value of electrolyte replacement after exercise. For example, if you sweat away 2 percent of your body weight during exercise, you reduce your electrolyte balance, and can put your heart under stress. Electrolytes must therefore be replaced. Rehydration with electrolyte sports drinks is standard procedure for athletes looking for muscle integrity after a workout. They know that dehydration severely limits performance and may contribute to heat stroke, organ damage, and possible death, if the fluids are not replaced. Electrolytes are the life-giving force lost in the dehydration process that account for the risk factor. It is essential to choose a sports drink or a supplement that provides you the basic elements — minerals that form electrolytes.

The Hunzas' of Pakistan, and the Vilcabambas tribe of Ecuador, live extraordinarily long, healthy lives. This is attributed to the fact that their home is in a mountainous area and their drinking sources contain highly mineralized and electrically charged water. The moose that appeared in the opening credits of the popular television show, Northern Exposure, died before his time. They attributed his death to a mineral deficiency because he was fed "civilized" food and given mineral deficient water. Mineral depleted soils are yielding mineral depleted food.[29]

Approximately four percent of the human body mass is composed of 21 macro and trace minerals that are essential for life. When mineral levels are insufficient to meet the demands of the body under emotional, physiological, and psychological stresses such as during physical activity, the result will most likely be a substandard level of performance. For athletes or weekend exercisers, this increases the risk of serious injury and reduces the recovery rate after strenuous work or exercise. Most of us are not ingesting sufficient amounts of minerals because our food and water

---

[29] *Variations in Mineral Content of Vegetables,* Acres, USA, March 1977.

is mineral deficient. To compound problems, athletes often induce low body weights by maintaining restrictive diets which do not contain the variety of foods needed for ingesting a wide range of minerals. Certain foods or drinks can actually create mineral deficiency. For example, drinks (carbonated) containing high levels of phosphorus cause the phosphorus to bind with calcium and move it out of the body. Calcium loss also increases following the consumption of either white sugar, salt, or caffeine. Therefore, carbonated drinks used for rehydration, containing these ingredients, should be avoided.

• *Is more better?*

Sports drinks and supplement manufacturers who claim their electrolyte-forming trace minerals facilitate proper rehydration may be only partially correct. Trace minerals work in combination to provide the proper environment for electrolyte formation and maximum absorption. According Dr. Gerald Olarsch, N.D., to *few* trace-minerals in a drink are unable to form the proper electrolyte balance to enter the cell and maximize rehydration. Only certain minerals will form electrolytes. For example, iron won't form electrolytes, but drinking electrolytes creates an electromagnetic energy in the body that will pull iron out from food and out of the blood into the cells.[30]

Too *many* trace-minerals in combination can actually prevent electrolyte formation. Minerals can compete with one another for absorption, especially if too much of one is available and not enough of others.[31] More is not necessarily better. The body utilizes only what it needs and the rest becomes very expensive toilet water. Many supplements contain fifty or more minerals, or so the label claims. Don't be fooled. More is not necessarily better. The body has the ability to use the trace elements as a key to unlock the rest of the minerals from the foods. By taking seventy minerals every day, you may just be unbalancing your body to the extent havoc

---

[30] Yarrow, David, *Fire in the Water*, Nature's Publishing, Ltd., 1999.
[31] ibid.

will be created. The proper combination of trace minerals are necessary for maximum hydration, and to provide the benefits sought.

• _Key minerals for supplementation:_

•**Boron**. Essential for plants, boron is a catalytic trace element that is suspected to play a role in the prevention and treatment of osteoporosis as it aids in the retention of calcium and magnesium in the bones. Studies indicate that boron improves the production of antibodies that help fight infection and markedly decreases peak secretion of insulin from the pancreas. The way in which boron acts in the body is not known, but a deficiency has proven to cause abnormal bone formation.

•**Calcium**.This is the most common mineral in the body. Adequate intakes of this mineral are an important determinant of bone health and risk of fracture. Calcium also carries an electric charge during an action potential across membranes and acts as an intracellular regulator and as a cofactor of enzymes and regulatory proteins.[32] Dietary recommendations set by the 1997 National Academy of Science Panel on Calcium and Related Nutrients are 1300 mg/day for children 9-18 years of age, 100 mg/day for those 19-50, and 1200 mg/day for those over 51. The most recent research shows that a proper balance of 1:1 should be maintained with magnesium for homeostasis in the body.[33] The form of calcium supplementation should be specified. For example, calcium carbonate is common blackboard chalk and cannot be adequately absorbed by the body. A better choice would be calcium citrate or calcium aspartate.[34]

•**Chloride**. As a natural salt of the mineral chlorine, chloride works with sodium and potassium to help in maintaining proper pH balance, healthy nerve and muscle function. It also contributes to

---

[32] Matkovic, Viliir, M.D., Ph.D., Connie Weaver, Ph.D., "Calcium," American Society for Nutritional Sciences, www.nutrition.org.

[33] Peiper, Howard, _Naturopathic Secrets for Building Better Bones_, Nature's Publishing Group, 2001.

[34] Martlew, Gillian, N.D., _Electrolytes The Spark of Life_, 1998 revised & updated, Nature's Publishing, Murdock FL.

digestion and waste elimination. Chloride should not be confused with the chemical chlorine used in water treatment. This chemical, when combined with waste in the digestive tract converts to trihalomethanes, a potential carcinogen. A diet of unprocessed foods provides more than enough dietary chloride.

•**Chromium**. Chromium is an essential nutrient required for normal sugar and fat metabolism. As an aid to glucose metabolism, chromium is essential to the regulation of blood sugar and fat metabolism. It protects against cardiovascular disease, diabetes, high cholesterol, and helps decrease body weight. Supplementation is essential if you eat white flour, milk and sugar as those foods steal chromium from the body and excrete it unused.

•**Cobalt**. As the key mineral in the vitamin B_{12} molecule, it is essential for proper nerve function and red blood cell formation.

•**Copper**. Copper is influential upon human health because it is a part of the body's enzymes, proteins that help biochemical reactions occur in all cells. Copper is required for the absorption and utilization of iron and the regeneration of blood. Copper and zinc together are crucial to the formation of collagen, connective tissues, and the protein fibers found in bone, cartilage, ligaments, dental tissues, and skin. Deficiency symptoms are similar to iron deficiency anemia, cardiac abnormalities, and elevated levels of serum cholesterol. Evidence exists that copper helps ease rheumatoid arthritis and other inflammatory diseases. Copper is utilized by most cells through enzymes involved in energy production, strengthening of connective tissue, and in brain neurotransmitters.

•**Germanium**. As a metallic trace mineral it is know to improve cellular oxygenation. It also fights pain, assists in immune system operation, act as an antioxidant, and improves stamina and endurance. Germanium acts as a carrier of oxygen to the cells.

•**Iodine**. This is a nonmetallic element that is converted to iodide in the gut and absorbed through the digestive tract. The thyroid gland needs this mineral to support metabolism, nerve and muscle function, physical and mental development. Deficiencies can lead to reduced brain function, growth stunting, apathy, impaired movement, speech, or hearing. Since soybeans, peanuts, cabbage, and turnips can block utilization of iodine, supplementation may be necessary in people who eat these foods.

•**Magnesium**. Not only does magnesium facilitate 300 fundamental enzymatic reactions, it also functions in the activation of amino acids and plays a key role in nerve transmissions and immune system operation. Numerous ATP-dependent reactions use magnesium as a cofactor.[35] This essential mineral enjoys a reciprocal relationship with calcium. In our muscles, calcium stimulates muscle fibers to tense up and contract whereas magnesium encourages the muscle fibers to loosen up and relax. Stored in the bones (60%) and muscles (40%), magnesium is called upon during exercise. Since bones do not release magnesium easily, the muscles are the target. The result may be cramps, irritability, or twitching. Supplemental calcium and magnesium in a 1:1 ratio are important to guard against this attack on our muscles.[36]

•**Manganese**. An essential element concentrated primarily in the bone, liver, pancreas, and brain. Manganese factors into cholesterol metabolism, normal skeletal growth and development. Manganese is responsible for transmitting nerve impulses to the muscles and for metabolism and RDA and DNA production. It is an important cofactor in the key enzymes of glucose metabolism. Lack of manganese has also been implicated in aggravating bone loss and porosity.

•**Molybdenum**. This is a component of a number of enzymes, including sulfite oxidase (deficiencies can cause metabolic disorders resulting in death at early age). It is required for nitrogen metabolism. It is essential in working with vitamin B_2 in the conversion of food to energy and is necessary for iron utilization. The Estimated Safe and Adequate Dietary Intakes of molybdenum in micrograms for adults are 75-250. Molybdenum deficiency is very rare, but is linked to an increased allergic reaction to sulfite food additives (such as additives to wine).

---

[35] Berning, Jacqueline R., Nelson Steen, S., *Nutrition for sport and exercise*, Aspen Publishers, Gaithersburg, MD, 1998.
[36] Peiper, Howard, *Naturopathic Secrets for Building Better Bones*, Nature's Publishing Group, 2001.

•**Potassium**. Potassium performs countless vital functions in the body supporting the nervous system, aiding in digestion, and providing the electrolyte charge to the cells. Most of the total body potassium is found in muscle tissue. Because of its link with the metabolizing, oxygen-consuming part of the body, a decline in total body potassium is usually interpreted as a loss of muscle mass. This is not necessarily the case, but muscle mass loss is the result of a catabolic protein wasting condition which reduces the total cell mass of the body.[37] Excess stress during exercise without proper nutrient components can facilitate this wasting condition. Low potassium in certain cases can lead to death.

•**Phosphorus**. As a key component of DNA, RNA, bones, and teeth, phosphorus plays an important role in energy metabolism of the cells affecting carbohydrates, fatty acids, and proteins. It is essential for bone formation and maintenance and stimulates muscle contraction. Deficiencies can appear as a general weakness, loss of appetite, bone pain, and susceptibility to fractures. Excesses in the bloodstream may promote calcium loss.

•**Selenium**. Shown to have a role in the detoxification of heavy metals, such as mercury, selenium plays a role in the production of antibodies in the immune system and may help prevent cancer and other degenerative diseases. Selenium protects cell membranes, cell nuclei and chromosomes from environmental damage. Preliminary studies suggest that it may have an anticancer effect on humans. Toxic levels of selenium can cause hair loss, nail problems, accelerated tooth decay and swelling of the fingers.

•**Silicon**. Shown to be necessary for normal growth and bone formation in animals, silicon has not been shown to be an essential element in human health. Growing evidence suggests it may have anti-aging properties because deficiencies of silicon apparently play a role in tissue degeneration.

•**Sodium**. Sodium acts together with potassium to maintain proper body water distribution and blood pressure, therefore being a primary ingredient necessary for rehydration. It is also important in

---

[37] Kehayias, Joseph J., Ph.D., Pierson, Richard N. Jr., M.D., American Society for Nutritional Sciences, 2001, www.nutrition.org.

maintaining the proper pH balance and to facilitate the transmission of nerve impulses. People with pronounced losses of sodium through heavy perspiration or diarrhea may experience decreased blood volume and a fall in blood pressure that could result in shock. Excessive amounts of sodium can lead to cardiac failure and liver disease. The Estimated Minimum Requirement of Health Persons from the National Academy of Sciences for adults is 500 milligrams per day.

•**Zinc**. No one can hope to be healthy without zinc. It is vital to the function of 90 enzymes that regulate dozens of bodily processes. It supports the immune system and fights infection, assists in chelating heavy metals from the body, improves vision, sexual potency and enhances the senses. Zinc also aids in cell respiration, bone development and growth, wound healing, and the regulation of heart rate and blood pressure. Together with copper is crucial to the formation of connective tissues and the protein fibers found in bone, cartilage, ligaments, dental tissues and skin. The average American diet is low in zinc, therefore zinc rich foods should be included in our menus.

Chapter 4: Sports drinks: A comparison.

Recently, there have been introduced to the market, a flurry of sports drinks, mixes, and electrolyte supplements. The marketing goals appear to be focused on rehydration and increased sports performance. While most companies producing the products seem to embrace the value of electrolytes, they may not have delivered the proper complement of ingredients for maximum electrolyte formation and absorption. Certain preservatives, artificial flavors and colored dyes, aspartame and sugar may add to the visual or taste appeal of the drink, but may not be user-friendly to the body.

In addition to its usefulness after exercise to replenish glycogen stores, sugar (fructose, dextrose, glucose, high fructose corn syrup, maltodextrin) is usually added as a carbohydrate to boost energy levels. While this may stimulate the body momentarily, minutes later the glycemic roller coaster sets in with associated compromise in body function. Muscle-testing (Kinesiology), used by chiropractors and natural medicine practitioners, reveals that sugar actually diffuses the body's ability to maintain muscle strength; therefore, it does not seem wise to use it when periods of strength are required. Sugar also creates cravings that generate a desire for more sweet drinks. In high quantities it also has been linked to diabetes. As blood glucose levels increase, people with diabetes are more at risk for heart disease.[38] Besides sugared drinks, there are other ways to get carbohydrates, such as energy bars, and complex carbohydrates found in apples, grapes, or peanuts. Furthermore, studies show that it may be the complex carbohydrates that support strength and endurance, rather than simple carbohydrates.[39]

The following pages include a chart of several sports drinks or drink supplements. Their electrolyte complement is revealed as well as calories and other ingredients. For instant rehydration we recommend pure electrolyte drinks with the proper complement of

---

[38] "Univ. Cambridge, U.K. study," British Med Jnl,vol. 322;15-18, Jan. 26, 2001.
[39] Martlew, Gillian, N.D., *"Electrolytes, The Spark of Life"*, 1998 revised & updated, Nature's Publishing, Murdock FL. $12.95 To order (800)-950-1929.

minerals. If you need a boost for short term energy or glycogen replacement, you may want to choose a drink containing less than 8 percent carbohydrates.

Note: Products may have different flavors and ingredients may vary, therefore not all ingredients may be listed. The intent of the chart is to acquaint you with the number of electrolytes in each drink for rehydration purposes, and the carbohydrates present for glucose replacement.

BRAND	Type	Calories	Carbohydrates and/or Sweetener	Electrolyte/Minerals	Ingredients Include
Alpha Lyte	electrolyte water drink	0	none	copper, iodine, manganese, zinc, potassium, cobalt, sodium, selenium, chromium, silica, boron	none
Athletic Edge	liquid electrolyte supplement	0	none	potassium, calcium, magnesium, chromium, selenium, zinc, platinum, germanium, sodium	none
Cytomax Grape	mix	160	32g carbs, fructose, dextrose	sodium, potassium, magnesium, chromium	calcium, ascorbic acid, vitamin A, beta-carotene, ginseng, quercetin, rutin, bioflavonoids
Dasani	water drink	0	none	sodium, potassium, magnesium	salt
Electroblast	effervescent electrolyte drink supplement	0	none	copper, iodine, boron, manganese, zinc, potassium, cobalt, sodium, selenium, chromium, silica, molybdenum plus replacement levels of sodium and potassium	stevia, vitamin C, sorbitol, natural lemon-lime flavor, citric acid
Gatorade Lemon-lime	drink	50	14g carbs, sucrose, glucose, fructose	sodium, potassium	salt, yellow 5

BRAND	Type	Calories	Carbohydrates and/or Sweetener	Electrolyte/Minerals	Ingredients Include
Hydra Fuel	mix	70	18g carbs, dextrose, fructose	sodium, potassium, chromium, chloride, phosphorus	calcium, iron
HydroLyte Citrus	mix	38	10g carbs, glucose	potassium, sodium, magnesium	calcium, ascorbic acid
Powerade Lemon-lime	drink	70	19g carbs, smaltodextrin, high fructose corn syrup	sodium, potassium	salt, yellow 5, ester of wood rosin
Power gel Tangerine	concentrated gel	110	28g carbs, maltodextrin, high fructose corn syrup	potassium, sodium	amino acids, salt, vitamins C & E, caffeine, kola nut extract, ginseng
Propel Fitness Water	drink	10	3G carbs, sucrose, sucralose, Acesulfame K	sodium, potassium, calcium	citric acid, vitamin C, E, B_5, B_6, B_{12}
Recharge Plus	drink	90	18g carbs, grape juice, lime juice	sodium, potassium, chromium	vitamin E, calcium, iron
Trace Lyte	electrolyte liquid supplement	0	none	copper, iodine, manganese, zinc, potassium, cobalt, sodium, selenium, chromium, silica, boron	none
Ultima	liquid	40	10g carbs, maltodextrin	70 ionic minerals incl. sodium, potassium	Ester C, Co-Q10, grapeseed, stevia

Chapter 5: **Other stuff in your sports drink.**

Water is good for rehydration. Water with electrolytes is better. Water with electrolytes and some carbohydrates is good for energy, but what else are they putting in those drinks? You have to be a dedicated label reader to know which ingredients in a food or drink product are beneficial to your body and which are harmful. Many ingredients in sports drinks come with a warning of health hazards if taken in quantity. Although one dose of a suspected carcinogen (such as an artificial dye) may not harm you, repeated use through ingestion of gallons of a sports drink may eventually cause symptoms.

Additives are designed to improve nutritional value, help with absorption, prevent spoilage, maintain freshness, act as a preservative, retard bacterial growth, provide cohesiveness, extend shelf life, enhance visual appearance, or act as a sweetener. Additives are not approved by the FDA when shown to be harmful in small amounts. But, if it only affects a small percentage of the population it can appear on the GRAS list (Generally Regarded As Safe) and allowed as an ingredient. Hopefully, you are not one of those statistical percentages that got sick.

Used as a deicing fluid for airplanes (considered hazardous material), propylene glycol is added to food and skin products to maintain texture and moisture as well as inhibit bacteria growth in the product. If you purchase a drum of propylene glycol, the supplier is required to furnish an MSDS (Material Safety Data Sheet), which says "Avoid Skin Contact" and gives a list of things to do if you do get it on your body or in your eyes. Propylene glycol has shown measurable toxicity to human cells in culture.[40] It has been reported to induce seizures in epileptics and cardio-respiratory arrest.[41] Reports also claim it inhibits the growth of the friendly bacteria in your intestines and decreases the amount of moisture in the intestinal tract leading to constipation and cancer. It is commonly used in drinks and most consider it safe because it is

---

[40] Bull Envir Contam Toxicol, Jan. 1987.
[41] Postgrad Med J, Aug. 1988.

included in small quantities. The cumulative effects of consumption have yet to be revealed.

Another chemical additive quite often found in sports drinks is PEG (polyethylene glycol). Sometimes used as a drug to induce mild diarrhea and cleanse the colon before surgery, it stays within the intestinal tract and is not absorbed. It is a water-soluble, waxy solid that is added to products to increase the freezing point. When given intravenously it tends to increase the ability of blood to clot, and if given rapidly causes clumping of cells and death from embolism.[42] Warnings from the MSDS labeling indicate that "if swallowed, give water and get medical assistance immediately. Avoid all unnecessary exposure and insure prompt removal from skin and clothing." Side effects are listed as nausea, bloating, cramps, vomiting, chills, and anal irritation. It also may interfere with drug effectiveness such as blood thinners, birth control pills, and anti-inflammatories.[43]

Most people are aware of the toxic side effects of artificial colors and flavors from coal tar derivatives such as Red #40, a possible carcinogen, and Yellow #6, which causes sensitivity to viruses and has caused death to animals, yet these are commonly used in sports drinks. Cochineal extract or Carmine Dye is a color additive used in food, drinks such as cola, cosmetics, and to dye fibers red. It is made of the ground up female cochineal bugs from Central and South America. University of Michigan allergist, James Baldwin, M.D., confirmed cochineal extract triggered life-threatening anaphylactic shock in some people.

Aspartame is a very popular sugar substitute, having very adverse effects on the human body. Aspartame comes with a list of potential side effects with the most profound being the possible detrimental effect on the neurotransmitters in the brain.[44] Headaches are a common side effect of aspartame (sometimes camouflaged as

---

[42] Smyth, H.F. Jr., Carpenter C.P., Weil C.S., (1950), J. Amer. Pharm. Assoc. Sci. Ed. 39. 349-354.

[43] Jackson Gastroenterology, "Polyethylene Glycol," July 1998, www.gicare.com.

[44] Nash Stoddard, Mary; Sweet but Deadly, Partners, June, 1998.

phenylalanine on the label). Other symptoms may be joint pain, depression, anxiety attacks, slurred speech, cramps, vertigo and dizziness. Scientific studies performed on aspartame to establish its safety prior to FDA approval, revealed brain tumors and grand mal seizures in rats during the studies. When exposed to heat, aspartame breaks down into toxic methyl alcohol.[45] This can occur during hot summer temperatures inside uncooled warehouses where diet drinks are stored and drinking them may cause recurrent headaches, mental aberrations, seizures, and suicidal tendencies. It has been implicated in Parkinson's disease and as a contributor to Alzheimer's.[46] Aspartame may not affect all users in the same way, although side effects may be difficult to pinpoint as being a result of using this common sweetener.

Another new sweetener is Acesulfame K. This is becoming more prevalent in some sports drinks. Tests show that the additive causes cancer in animals, which means it may increase cancer in humans.[47] Sucralose is a newer artificial sweetener produced by chlorinating sugar. Few human studies have been conducted as to the safety of this product but results in animals show a negative effect on the thymus gland, enlarged liver and kidneys, decreased red blood cell count, aborted pregnancy, and diarrhea. Although the manufacturer claims that sucralose passes through the body unabsorbed, tests reported from the Japanese Food Sanitation Council show that 40 percent of ingested sucralose is absorbed.

Many sports drinks include favorable ingredients such as vitamins (C, B, D), herbs (stevia, rhodiola) and other beneficial ingredients such as antioxidants (grape seed extract, pycnogenol, rhododendron caucasicum, Co-enzyme Q_{10}). Sweeteners may be added as carbohydrates and include glucose, fructose, high fructose corn syrup, sugar, maltodextrin, and dextrose.

---

[45] Dadd, Debra Lynn, *Nontoxic, Natural & Earthwise*, Jeremy P. Tarcher, Inc. Los Angeles, 1990.

[46] Blaylock, Richard, *Excitotoxins: The Taste that Kills,* Health Press, Santa Fe, NM, 1997.

[47] "Food Additives to Avoid," Center for Science in the Public Interest, 1875 Conn. Ave. NW Ste. 300, Wash. DC 20009; www.cspinet.org.

Chapter 6: Benefits:
Electrolyte and mineral replacement.

Electrolyte replacement is critical for sports enthusiasts. High volume oxygen intake during athletic exertion oxidizes blood cells faster than normal and increases the change of anemia. Electrolytes are the ultimate oxygenator of all living cells through a process known as bio-oxygenation. The building of muscle and the production of energy draws on chromium, acting as a cofactor to insulin. It also promotes the entrance of glucose and amino acids into the cells to make muscle. A loss of potassium can cause dizzy spells or lightheadedness, especially during exertion in hot weather. The proper complement of minerals forming a proper electrolyte drink or supplement, when taken daily, may help to provide the following benefits:

- Promotes faster recovery from injury stress or strenuous exercise.
- Quickly heightens concentration and alertness.
- Supports neurotransmitter function in the brain.
- IncreaseS oxygen uptake at the cellular level.
- Dramatically boosts energy levels.
- Strengthens the immune system.
- Helps to strengthen hair and restore pigmentation.
- Assists in peristaltic action of bowel muscles.
- Rapidly helps kill infectious bacteria, viruses, yeast, fungi, and parasites without harming beneficial microorganism.
- Improves digestion (especially if taken with plant enzymes).
- Raises osmotic pressure level of cells to keep them strong.
- Increases body enzyme production.
- Helps keep the body's homeostasis balance.
- Aids in efficient removal of toxic body acids.
- Enhances uptake of vitamins, macro minerals, proteins and other essential nutrients from natural food sources or dietary supplements.
- Helps to reestablish healthy pH levels.

• *The importance of minerals.*

Minerals serve three roles: a) they provide structure in forming bones and teeth, b) they help maintain normal heart rhythm, muscle contractility, neural conductivity, and acid-base balance, and c) they help regulate cellular metabolism by becoming part of enzymes and hormones that modulate cellular activity. Minerals cannot be made in the body and must be obtained from our diets. Dr. Firman Bear of the Department of Agricultural Chemistry at Rutgers University tested the mineral levels of 204 samples of vegetables and discovered that the foods most of us are eating are not what we think they are.

According to the U.S. Senate Document #264, (1936), "It is bad news to learn from our leading authorities that 99 percent of the American people are deficient in minerals." It continues, "Our physical well-being is more directly dependent upon the minerals we take into our systems than upon the calories or vitamins, or upon the precise proportion of starch, protein or carbohydrates we consume?" A marked deficiency in any one of the more important minerals actually results in disease, particularly, degenerative disease. This condition hasn't changed much in the last sixty years.

It seems that modern agricultural methods and acid rain have washed the minerals from our growing soil.[48] Even organic gardeners are not immune to this problem. They may not feed their plants pesticides or chemical fertilizers, but the nutrient rich topsoil (which has decreased from three feet 200 years ago to only 6 inches today), cannot sustain healthy plants. The plants are hungry, so in a frenzy to munch on anything in the ground that will nourish them, they take up the pesticide residue, fertilizers, inorganic aluminum (from the acid rain) and other noxious metals which become part of the food chain.

Electrolyte replacement drinks offer you mineral supplementation, primarily sodium and potassium, commonly lost during

---

[48] "Eden or Ice Age," Remineralize The Earth Magazine, Spring 1996. Gor subscription: 152 South St., Northampton, MA 01060-4021, (413)-586-4429, E-mail: ReminEarth@aol.com.

exercise. These are not the only minerals your body needs to replace. Since many of us drink bottled or filtered water, you may become mineral deficient. Minerals, naturally occurring in the water, are commonly eliminated through many of the filtration systems needed for purification. This means that it is unlikely you will get the necessary amounts of minerals your body needs, and in the proper ratio.

Stress also affects your mineral balance as well as laxatives or antacids or medicinal drugs.[49] The following chart reveals how some popular drugs affect your mineral balance.

DRUG	MINERAL AFFECTED
Antifungal	Potassium
Antacids	Calcium, magnesium, phosphorous
Aspirin	Calcium, magnesium, phosphorus, potassium
Diuretics	Calcium, chromium, iodine, magnesium, sodium, zinc, phosphorus, potassium
Cholesterol medications	Iron
Penicillins	Magnesium, potassium
Ulcer medications	Iron, potassium

Toxic metals from environmental pollution such as lead, mercury, and cadmium can interfere with mineral absorption and increase mineral excretion. Even taking vitamins unknowingly can upset the mineral balance. Vitamin C is required for iron absorption, but in excess amounts can cause a copper deficiency. Vitamin D enhances calcium absorption, but in excess amounts can produce a magnesium deficiency. When the mineral balance is upset, our immune systems go on vacation and we get more illnesses and more stressed out, causing the leaching of more minerals. It's a merry-go-round effect that we have to stop.

---

[49] Reproduced from the book *Electrolytes The Spark of Life* by Gillian Martlew, N.D., Nature's Publishing, Ltd. 1994.

The following list will tell you which minerals can contribute to symptoms of a specific illness. Oxygen is mentioned because it is normally supplied to the cells by electrolytes.

Illnesses	Mineral deficiency
A.D.D./A.D.H.D.	Chromium, Magnesium, Zinc, Manganese, Copper
Age spots	Selenium
Aging skin	Selenium
Alopecia (hair loss)	Zinc
Alzheimer's disease	Selenium
Anemia	Copper, Iron, Selenium, Zinc
Aneurysms	Copper
Anorexia	Magnesium
Arterial calcification	Magnesium
Arthritis	Copper, Selenium,
Asthma	Magnesium, Manganese
Behavior (violent)	Copper
Birth defects (congenital)	Zinc
Birth weight low	Selenium
Blood cholesterol elevated	Chromium
Blood sugar low	Chromium
Blood triglycerides elevated	Chromium
Body odor (severe)	Zinc
Bone Spurs	Calcium
Bones (weak)	Calcium
Brain defects	Zinc
Calcium deposits	Calcium
Cancer	Selenium, Lack of oxygen
Carpal Tunnel Syndrome	Manganese
Cataracts	Chromium
Cholesterol (high)	Copper
Chronic Fatigue	Lack of oxygen
Convulsions	Magnesium, Manganese
Coronary blood vessel disease	Chromium

Cramping	Magnesium, Calcium
Depression	Chromium, Lithium, Zinc, Magnesium
Diabetes	Chromium
Diarrhea	Zinc
Estrogen (low)	Calcium
Eyelids sagging	Copper
Eyes (small)	Zinc
Fatigue	Iron, Selenium
Gastrointestinal disturbances	Magnesium
Hair (frizzy)	Zinc
Hair (gray)	Copper
Hair (white)	Copper
Hair (dry, brittle)	Copper
Heartbeat (irregular)	Selenium
Heart palpitations	Selenium
Heart weakness	Selenium
Hyperactivity	Chromium
Impaired growth	Chromium
Impotence	Chromium, Zinc
Infertility	Chromium, Selenium, Zinc
Insomnia	Calcium
Kidney Stones	Calcium
Learning Disabilities	Chromium, Copper
Liver cirrhosis	Copper, Selenium
Liver damage	Selenium
Loss of libido	Manganese
Lower Back Problems	Calcium
Low blood sugar	Copper
Manic depression	Chromium, Lithium
Menstrual difficulties	Iodine
Menstrual migraines	Magnesium
Muscle Cramps	Calcium
Muscular weakness	Selenium
Nervous system degeneration	Copper

Neuromuscular problems	Magnesium
Osteoporosis	Calcium, Magnesium
Panic attacks	Calcium
PMS	Calcium
Prediabetes	Chromium
Prostate enlargement	Zinc
Reproductive failure	Copper
Rheumatoid arthritis	Lack of oxygen
Scoliosis	Selenium
Sense of smell, taste (loss of)	Zinc
Sexual maturation delayed	Zinc
SIDS	Selenium
Toxic Shock syndrome	Lack of oxygen
Tremors	Magnesium
Varicose Veins	Copper
Vertigo	Magnesium

• *Trace Minerals*

Minerals are sometimes referred to as trace elements because they exist in such tiny, yet powerful amounts in the body, and are needed for overall mental and physical functioning. Trace-minerals are those minerals that are considered to be required in our diets in amounts of less than 100 milligrams per day. [50]

The consensus among experts is that the minerals most vital to humans are electrolytes, elements that in solution form positive and negative electrically charged particles (ions) that will conduct electricity. The ratio of these elements to one another is a determining factor in good health. The body has a magnificent ability (homeostasis) to adjust and rearrange materials according to specific requirements as long as they have the proper building blocks (minerals & enzymes) to work with. Dr. Bernard Jensen writes, "We cannot heal a person through symptomatic relief. We must go

---

[50] Heinrich, Elmer G., *The Root of All Disease*, TRC, 2000.

to the root of the problem — to the cell itself — where electrolytes are at work giving life. It is here that real healing can begin." [51]

Seven major minerals occur in the body and are needed in large amounts: Calcium, potassium, sulfur, sodium, chlorine, phosphorus, and magnesium. Trace minerals exist in very tiny amounts, but they are a key constituent in maintaining homeostasis in the body. This "natural regulator" is your body's auto-regulatory mechanism and it works to keep your body in balance — or in a state of homeostasis. Why are trace elements considered essential? When a deficiency in the intake of trace minerals occurs, results consistently show an impairment of specific bodily functions (i.e. kidney stones may be a result of calcium deficiency). With dietary changes, along with supplemental trace minerals, the pain and degenerative processes of illness may be arrested. The key to this lies in the fact that trace minerals, dissolved in water, are far more bioavailable than those present in food and thus are effective when included in an electrolyte sports drink.

Trace minerals support the health of our glands and the production of the hormones that control calcium's use in the body. Therefore, they should be factored in as a key consideration to reduce the risk of osteoporosis. One of the first signals of restoring trace mineral levels in the body is improved digestion. The acid/alkaline (pH) balance is stabilized, resulting in the production of digestive acids and enzymes. Trace mineral-forming electrolytes aid in the conversion of proteins to their component amino acids, necessary during athletic endeavors. Properly formed electrolytes help to chelate toxic and *inorganic* minerals out of the body before they cause damage. Electrolytes assist in the absorption of *organic* minerals into the cells where the body can use them.

Trace minerals, when abundant in water, enhance absorption and utilization of minerals in food. Bear in mind that as we mentioned earlier, foods are becoming mineral deficient because of poor soil conditions.

---

[51] Excerpted from "Are Minerals The Missing Link?," Issue 13, Health Science Newsletter, N. Warsaw St., Ursa, IL 62376.

Food Sources of some common minerals:

- Calcium: sea vegetables, dark leafy greens, dandelion greens, broccoli, salmon, sardines, dairy products
- Chromium: nutritional yeast, potatoes with skin on, most vegetables, whole grain bread, cheese, chicken, fruit, seafood
- Copper: grains, chocolate, nuts, meats, shellfish
- Germanium: garlic, shiitake mushrooms, onions, ginseng
- Iodine: iodized salt, grain, some dairy products, seaweeds
- Magnesium: sprouted soy products, buckwheat, nuts, kidney beans, whole wheat flour, banana, beet greens, avocado, peanut butter, potato, oatmeal
- Manganese: pecans, peanuts, pineapple, oatmeal, beans, rice, spinach, sweet potato, wheat
- Molybdenum: legumes, whole grains, milk, leafy vegetables
- Phosphorus: meat, poultry, eggs, fish, nuts, whole grains, dairy
- Potassium: potato, avocado, raisins, sardines, flounder, salmon, cod, haddock, orange juice, winter squash, bananas, tomato, turkey, chicken, milk
- Selenium: meat, fish, grains, Brazil nuts, garlic, eggs,
- Sodium: salt, soy sauce, processed cheeses, canned soups, etc.
- Zinc: Beef, chicken liver, turkey, pumpkin seeds, cheese, oysters, sunflower seeds, oats, peanuts, peas, chick peas, lentils, shrimp

Foods that block or reduce mineral absorption:

- Refined foods, sugar, dark drinks (cola, coffee, hot chocolate), white flour, caffeine (leaches out potassium)

Before implementing any nutrient regimen you should find out where you stand with respect to your mineral balance. We have employed hair analysis procedures as well as cellular microscopy to determine the state of our cells. In both instances, by retesting a year after taking the electrolytes, we saw visible changes. These results indicate our constitutions were much improved and our cellular structure was more balanced. Please, for your sake and for the sake of your children and your pets (yes, they need minerals and electrolytes too), take this information to heart.

• *Mineral Supplementation — pick the right one.*

You can think of the actual form of mineral found in supplements, as coming in sizes: Colloidal is the largest, chelated smaller, ionic smaller yet, and ionic when dispersed in water becomes even smaller (crystalloid).

Colloidal minerals are suspended in a liquid such as the blood. They are too large to become dissolved. In order to get into the cell membrane where minerals do their work, they must be dissolved in a solution. To be absorbed through the cell wall, a mineral must be smaller than the colloidal mineral form. Colloidal particles will readily pass through a filter paper, but they are too large to pass through a living membrane.[52] Colloidal particles cannot undergo osmosis. This means colloidal minerals are unable to get inside the cell. It may become debris floating around in the bloodstream looking for a nook or cranny to call home. These deposits may accumulate into arthritic conditions or kidney stones. Colloidal minerals were designed by nature to nourish plants *after being broken down by organisms in the soil.* Even the plants won't use this large form of minerals unless they are munched up by critters in the dirt so don't try to give your old bottles of colloidal minerals to your houseplants.

A plant is able to utilize minerals through chelation, which converts the minerals into a form that is more assimilated by humans and animals and therefore more beneficial. Ionic minerals are smaller than colloidal or chelated and have an even better chance of getting into the cell. When you put these ionic minerals into water they will break down into a solution known as crystalloid, which is highly absorbable. Ionic minerals, which may be considered inorganic by some standards, are actually pure living minerals. Minerals must get into the cell to benefit the body. The water-dispersed form of ionic minerals is assimilated 100 percent by the body and gets into the cell, bypassing the digestive system and providing the electrical energy necessary to run the organism.

---

[52] *Say No To Collodial Minerals*, Sunset Adventures Press, Issue 4, June 1996.

• *Individual minerals or combination supplements?*

For those of us who are not chemists, we cannot possibly determine exactly what individual minerals do when they meet other minerals. Some compete with others for absorption, especially if too much of one is available and not enough of others. For example, too much zinc can unbalance copper and iron levels. Large amounts of calcium (2000 mg.) reduce absorption of magnesium, zinc, phosphorus and manganese. So how can you possibly determine which minerals to take, when, and in what dosages?

Our suggestion is to leave it to the experts who have to, by law, determine the safety of supplements. They have created products that they claim include the minerals in proper balance. The researchers, chemists, and manufacturers normally are conscientious and have your best interest at heart, but sometimes they take a wrong tack. Many supplements and drugs have been released to market, and several years down the road proved to be dangerous. Sports drink manufacturers may be too anxious to provide a product and can overlook the need for properly designed electrolyte or carbohydrate replacements. It is up to the consumer to increase their awareness of what is being consumed, and gain the knowledge to properly choose the fuel they need for the task at hand.

Resource Directory

SYN-R-GY™ The Ultimate in Athletic Formulas. Decades of scientific research combined with the purest adaptogens and botanicals sourced from around the globe prove that by adding SYN-R-GY™ to an athletic program may make the difference between a workout and a record. SYN-R-GY™ is the only product in the world proven to dramatically increase muscle size, mental well being and overall endurance at the same time. The large "R" in SYN-R-GY™ stands for Rhaponticum carthamoides, a natural anabolic steroid (without undesirable side-effects) that can burn fat into muscle up to 20 times faster than working out alone. Combining Rhaponticum with the other well-researched adaptogens such as Siberian Ginseng, Rhodiola rosea, Aralia mandjurica, and Schizandra extract may give the average person an incredible edge in competition and quite possibly turn an athlete into an Olympian. AMERIDEN™ International, LLC, P.O. Box 1870, Fallbrook, CA 92088 (888) 405-3336 www.ameriden.com

ELECTROBLAST™ A lemon-lime flavored effervescent tablet in a portable formulation of essential electrolytes. ELECTROBLAST™ provides eleven trace-minerals including sodium and potassium, plus molybdenum, and vitamin C. It makes an ideal electrolyte-replacement drink when dissolved into 8-10 oz. water. Used in competitive sports, at the fitness center, by physically active people, air travelers, and those living or working in dry environments, ELECTROBLAST™ is the most convenient way to add minerals to your diet. LJB PIPER, LLC, P.O. Box 1454, Lakeville, CT, 06039 (888) 217-7233 www.electroblast.com

LIQUID CRYSTALLOID ELECTROLYTE MINERALS.

Trace-Lyte ™ is a crystalloid (smallest form) electrolyte formula that helps keep cells strong, balance pH, facilitate removal of toxins, and provide the body's life force. As an aid to restoration of body cellular osmotic equilibrium, pH balance and electrical potential, this liquid supplement provides 11 essential trace minerals needed to form electrolytes, including organic copper, iodine, manganese, zinc, potassium, cobalt, sodium, selenium, chromium, silica, and boron. NATURE'S PATH, INC., PO Box 7862, Venice, FL 34287-7862 (800) 326-5772. www.naturespathinc.com

Other Books to Read.

The All-natural High Performance Diet	$7.95 US
Improve your physical, mental, sexual performance.	$11.95 CA
Overcoming Senior Moments	$7.95 US
Increase your brain power.	$11.95 CA
Crystalloid Electrolytes (Audio tape)	$9.95 US
Your body's energy source for the new millennium.	$14.95 CA
Nutritional Leverage for Great Golf	$9.95 US
Improve your score on the back nine.	$14.95 CA
Fitness for Golfer's Handbook	$14.95 US
Exercise tips for great golfing.	$19.95 CA
Eliminating Pilot Error	$7.95 US
Fitness tips for pilots.	$11.95 CA
A Doctor in Your Suitcase	$7.95 US
Natural treatments for travel ills.	$11.95 CA
The Brain Train	$4.95 US
Improve childrens' thinking power.	$7.95 CA

Order Line: (888) 628-8731